Holistic Brain Health (6 Cornerstones of a Healthy Brain)

Danny Nandy

Published by Mystic Media Publishing, 2021.

HOLISTIC BRAIN HEALTH (6 CORNERSTONES OF A HEALTHY BRAIN)

First edition. December 16, 2021.

Copyright © 2021 Danny Nandy.

ISBN: 979-8215337066

Written by Danny Nandy.

Table of Contents

The Human Brain - A Fascinating Mystery

The human brain is a fascinating machine, a miracle really that is the central command center of all that gives us life and makes us human.

> *"The study of the mind and brain is the last frontier in science. Although the field has made enormous progress over the past several decades, understanding of the basic principles of thought and brain function are still far more unknown than known," said Michael Tarr, co-director of the CNBC and the Cowan Professor of Cognitive Neuroscience. "Personally, I think that unraveling how the mind and brain work is a significant step in understanding what makes humans human."*

As we go through life, from growing within our mother's womb, to birth, to infancy and into our older years, our brains manage our physical movements, thoughts, learning, emotions and everything in between.

It's fascinating how such a fragile organ, can be so very powerful at the same time.

Brain health is not often considered as people strive to look after their physical health, but it should be an important consideration in keeping it healthy, thriving and serving you until your dying day.

23 Fascinating Brain Facts

> "Our minds influence the key activity of the brain, which then influences everything; perception, cognition, thoughts and feelings, personal relationships; they're all a projection of you"
>
> — Deepak Chopra

According to Cleveland Clinic's Healthy Brain Website

➤ Your brain processes about 70,000 thoughts each and every day

➤ Your brain works 24 hours a day, 7 days a week

➤ The human brain continues to grow and change throughout life

➤ The human brain, while so powerful and efficient, is very gelatin like with a tofu-like consistency, and it's very fragile

➤ Psychology Today reports that 70% of the estimated 70,000 thoughts people have each day are negative.

➤ The human brain is the most powerful supercomputer known to man

➤ You can power a small light bulb with the electricity created in the brain

➤ The human brain requires 20% of the entire body's blood flow and the human brain holds over 400 miles of blood vessels

➤ Medical science and researchers say that there is more that is unknown about the brain than what is known

➤ Without a brain, there is no awareness of self or the world

➤ The human brain is the most powerful learning tool in the world. It is an intricate and complex network comprised of 100 billion neurons that meet at over 500 trillion synapses that travel 300 miles per hour

➤ Signals that travel through the neuronal brain network form a complex highway that is the basis of feelings, thoughts, and memories

➤ Throughout a human life, the brain codes memories, skills, thoughts, emotions and a sense of self by creating patterns of activity

➤ The adult human brain weighs about 3 pounds, certainly not the heaviest in the animal kingdom, as the sperm whale's brain weighs 17-pounds

➤ The size of a brain does not determine its performance or smartness level, so bigger is not better

➤ Like the human body, the brain ages by shrinking in size, slowing in speed and becoming less adaptable to change

➤ When something new is learned the structure of the brain changes and new brain connections are created with each new memory

➤ While often attributed to the heart, brain imaging studies show that human emotions actually originate in the brain

➤ Loss of oxygen to the brain for even 5 minutes can cause serious and permanent brain damage

➤ Music triggers dopamine and pleasure centers in the brain, just like sex and drugs

➤ 25% of all cholesterol found in the human body lives inside the brain, and it is a critical element of each and every brain cell. Insufficient cholesterol within the brain causes cell death (Ingemar Björkhem, Steve Meaney, Arteriosclerosis, Thrombosis, and Vascular Biology)

➤ The brain consists of 73% water (According to H.H. Mitchell, Journal of Biological Chemistry 158). Dehydration at only 2% will negatively affect memory, attention and other key cognitive skills. Only 90 minutes of sweating can cause a temporary shrinkage of the brain that is equivalent to one year of aging

➤ Ever get drunk and can't remember the night? This is because the brain cannot form memories while drunk

Brain Structure

> "The brain is a wonderful organ; it starts working the moment you get up in the morning and does not stop until you get into the office"
>
> – Robert Frost

According to Bryn Mawr University, the body's central nervous system, the CNS consists of the brain and spinal cord. The peripheral nervous system, or PNS consists of nerves.

The CNS and PNS are the two parts of the nervous system that is the body's decision and communication center.

Everything you do, from standing up, to blinking, to making a decision, having an emotion, or solving a complex mathematical equation and everything in between is controlled by your nervous system.

Sensory nerves gather data interpreted from the environment, send that data to the spinal cord, which sends messages to your brain, which then reacts accordingly.

Neurons send instructions from the brain to the body. The entire system is a highly efficient superhighway that sends an enormous amount of messages to and from the brain every second of everyday.

Parts Of The Brain

Forebrain

· Cerebrum

· Thalamus
· Hypothalamus

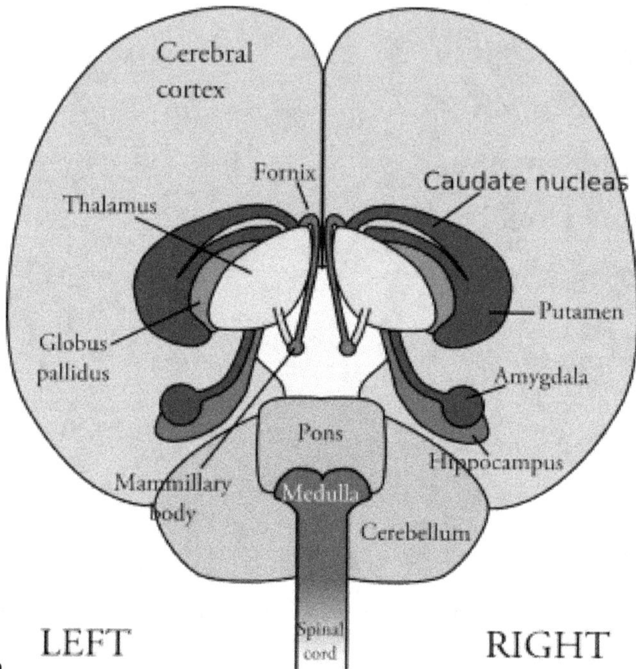

Brain Stem

· **Midbrain**

- Tectum
- Tegmentum

· **Hindbrain**

- Cerebellum
- Pons
- Medulla

The Cerebrum

The cerebrum, also referred to as the frontal cortex is the largest part of the brain.

This is a principle area located at the front of the skull and consists of two different hemispheres.

It is within the cerebrum that higher thought and action functions take place, along with integration of complicated sensory and neural functions and voluntary body activity.

The cerebral cortex is divided into four different sections known as lobes

Frontal Lobe

- Planning
- Reasoning
- Movement
- Emotions
- Problem solving
- And some speech function

Parietal Lobe

- Perception of stimuli
- Orientation
- Movement
- Recognition

Occipital Lobe

- Vision and visual processing

Temporal Lobe

- Memory
- Speech
- Perception
- Auditory functions

The cortex is the "grey matter," the outer part of the brain, which does not start to develop until after a baby is born. The cortex is responsible for the more sophisticated of our mental processes like abstract thought and introspection. The more wrinkled it is, the better.

> " Biology gives you a brain. Life turns it into a mind"
>
> – Jeffrey

The highly wrinkled design of the cerebral cortex or cortical folding (gyrencephalization) allows for an increased surface area that facilitates a mass amount of neurons, which make it so highly efficient.

- The frontal cortex is where thoughts are generated, and problem solving and planning takes place.

- It also interprets various sensations and signals that come from within your body and smells, sounds and sights from the outside world.

- The frontal cortex also helps to form and store memories, and controls all your voluntary movements.

The Cerebellum

The cerebellum, which is referred to as the "little brain" is also highly folded and consists of two hemispheres.

The cerebellum regulates

- Movement
- Posture

· Balance
· Coordination

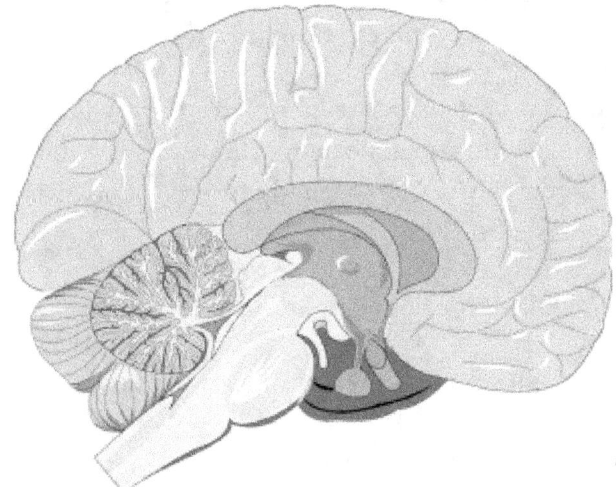

The Limbic System

· Limbic System ("emotional brain")
· Thalamus
· Hypothalamus
· Amygdala
· Hippocampus

Brain Stem

The brain stem lies underneath the limbic system and regulates breathing, blood pressure and other vital functions within the body.

Parts Of The Brain Stem

· Medulla
· Pons
· Midbrain

Two Hemispheres

According to Wikipedia, the brain is divided into two hemispheres, the left, and the right. While both hemispheres are symmetrical, and experts readily admit they do not know enough about how the two sides differ, studies have found that each side functions slightly different from the other.

· The right hemisphere has been associated with creativity while the left with logical thinking skills, though experts admit this is a much too simplistic view as brain structure is highly complex and many variables play a role in its functions

· The left hemisphere regulates the body's right side (movement)

· The right hemisphere regulates the body's left side (movement)

· Language areas are mostly on the left side

The Neuron Forest

According to the Alzheimer's Association, the brain's greatest work takes place within its individual cells.

There are about 100 billion nerve cells (neurons) in each adult brain that branch out and connect to more than 100 trillion points throughout the brain's landscape.

This network is called the neuron forest and it handles millions of signals that travel within each day to manage every single thing that your body does, including the formation of memories, moving your arm and the experience of emotions, and thinking.

According to The Scientist, *While the understanding of how neural" connections work is improving by leaps and bounds, the sheer numbers of neurons in the human brain (100 billion) and the complexity of the brain's wiring (100 trillion "connections) are daunting*

According to PubMed (National Institutes of Health), each neuron in the brain has a cell body and multiple extensions.

The shorter extensions are known as dendrites and they are the antennas of brain cells, receiving signals that they send to the cell body where they are then passed to the long extensions known as axons, which maybe up to a meter in length.

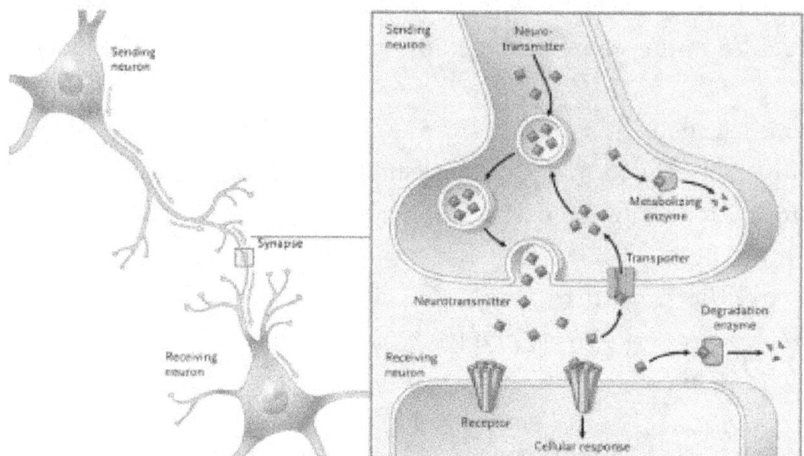

The brain's nerve cells connect to one another at areas known as synapses. Signals in the brain move in the form of a tiny electrical charge. When such a charge reaches a synapse it releases bursts of chemicals known as neurotransmitters, which then travel across the synapse to a receptor site and carry signals to other cells in the brain.

The receptor is actually the dictator of the neurotransmitter's effect. There are dozens of different neurotransmitters, all with their own functions and sets of actions.

Examples Of Neurotransmitter Actions

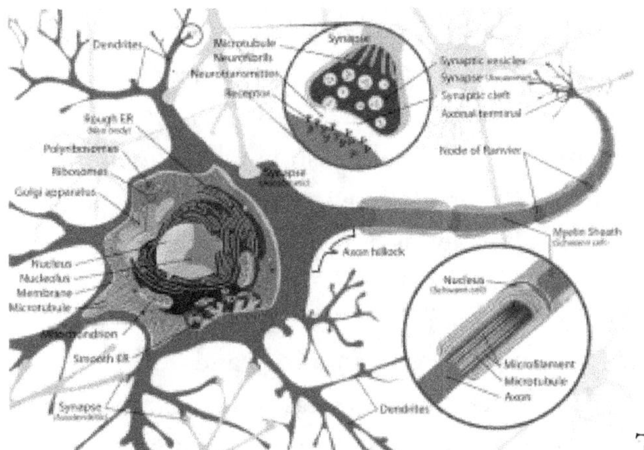

The topic of neurotransmission is a very complicated one, as it has many facets, actions and reactions as well as a complex chemistry that takes place in the brain, one of the reasons that neurologists and brain researchers spend years in school, however, here are some examples of the various actions of specific neurotransmitters.

- **Serotonin** regulates mood, emotions including depression and anxiety, memory, sleep, wakefulness and temperature regulation (New World Encyclopedia). Psychology Today reports that disruptions in serotonin is central to various types of depressive disorders, including, major depression.

- **Norepinephrine** regulates arousal (New World Encyclopedia)

- **Acetylcholine** regulates voluntary movement of the muscles (New World Encyclopedia)

- **According to Psychology Today,** dopamine supports the flow of information from other areas of the brain within the frontal lobes, where dopamine related disorders could result in a decline in neurocognitive function, including problem solving, attention and memory.

The death of dopamine neurons in the nigrostriatal pathway of the brain is the cause of Parkinson's disease that features a loss of ability to make smooth, controlled movements.

Dopamine is associated with the 'pleasure system' of the brain; as certain activities prompt its release yielding feelings of enjoyment that reinforce motivation to continue doing such activities. In fact, the firing of dopamine neurons can occur just at the thought or expectation of an upcoming pleasurable activity, regardless of whether it occurs or not. Brain scans show levels of dopamine released during orgasms similar to that when someone is on heroin.

Addictions, including cocaine, sex, gambling and others are significantly fueled by the effects dopamine has on the brain as the strong euphoric feelings and rewards elicited by the dopamine release motivates the user to continue, which eventually results in a loss of control. Psychosis and schizophrenia are strongly linked to disruptions and/or break downs in the dopamine system.

· **Glycine** regulates spinal reflexes and motor behavior (New World Encyclopedia)

· **Neuromodulators** regulate various types of sensory transmission, especially pain (New World Encyclopedia)

Brain Plasticity

> **FACT**
> **Forgetting is helpful for the brain as deleting unnecessary information promotes the retention of plasticity**

According to the Administration For Community Living, there is only one thing that is constant about the human brain and that is that it is always changing.

This phenomenon is known as "brain plasticity" and it occurs through different stages of life, through learning, experience and habits, Through everything we do the brain adapts, and grows new connections and repair those that are broken.

It is truly our knowledge, and experiences that keep the brain alive, developing, learning, and working to serve us.

Brain Changes Through Your Years

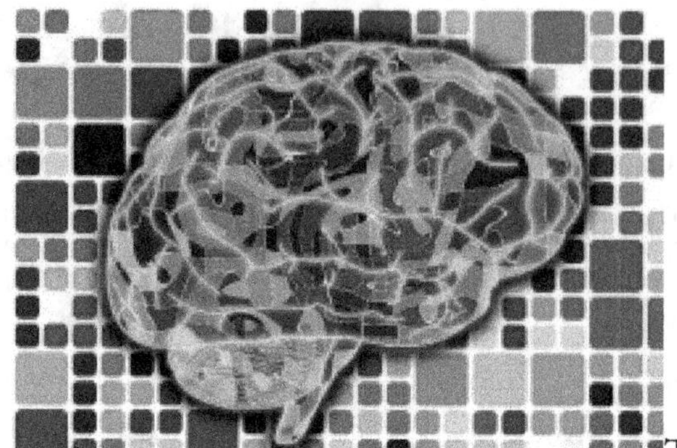

· The brain reaches 90% of adult size by age five as and cells become much more efficient at communicating with each other.

· Spatial understanding and language centers of the brain see dramatic growth between the ages of 5 and 10.

• By your 20s your brain's reasoning, planning and impulse control centers are fully formed.

• During this time, long-term memory and complex reasoning functions reach their peak, and creativity is believed to be at an all-time high

· The slow and gradual process of brain shrinking begins, as there is a slight decline in neurons.

· The beginning of the gradual age-related brain volume decline begins to show, this can affect the sharpness of memory and recollection.

· Reactions to complex stimuli may become slowed and take longer to perform.

· Typically, vocabulary, conceptual understanding, language functions, cognition, wisdom, and creativity remain strong.

· Often, people in their 50s begin to report memory failings, such as the inability to recall names of favorite songs, appointments and other data that was once much easier to retrieve. Memory distortion is another side-effect of aging. Stuart Zola, PhD, professor of psychiatry and behavioral sciences at the Emory School of Medicine and director of Yerkes National Primate Facility in Atlanta tells WebMD that, *"This is the phenomenon where as time passes our ability to accurately recall events becomes diminished—and the longer the period of time that passes between the event and trying to recall it, the greater the chance we're going to have some memory distortions and forgetting, sometimes time distortion causes us to forget the event totally."*

· Reasoning, knowledge, and problem solving can remain strong. Memory can remain strong, but many notice failure in retrieval of data that was once much easier to access.

· Cognitive processing speed may slow down as certain brain regions begin to shrink.

· For many people, reasoning, language functions, creativity, and procedural memories continue to stay sharp.

· For others, genetic factors, lifestyle choices, and general health will affect brain function with noticeable effects. At this stage, signs of brain dysfunction can occur, such as the onset of dementia, Alzheimer's, and other brain degenerative diseases. Symptoms should be addressed early with a qualified medical professional.

How The Brain Is Nourished

> **FACT**
> **The brain uses 20% of the total oxygen and blood in your body**

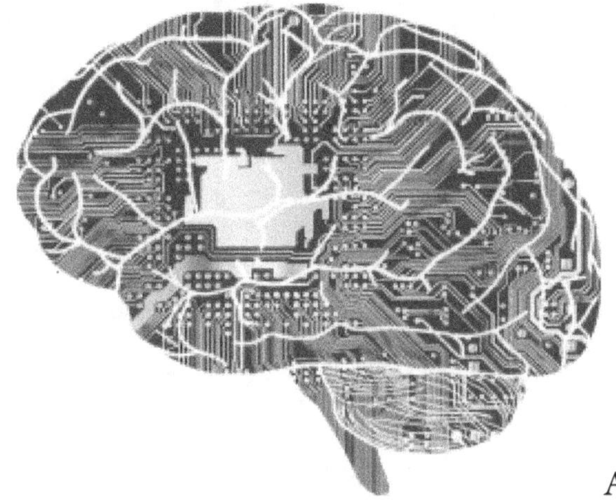

According to WebMD, the brain gets all its nourishment through a complex network superhighway of blood vessels, which is comprised of capillaries, arteries, and veins.

Each heartbeat results in arteries carrying around 20% to 25% of all the blood in your body to the brain, where billions of cells will use the oxygen and the fuel your blood brings.

The brain actually uses as much as 50% of the body's oxygen and fuel when you are in a state of deep concentration or thought.

12 Cornerstones Of Holistic Brain Health

Just as your lifestyle choices play a significant role for your physical health, they do as well for your brain and mental health.

Physical

"A man should keep his little brain attic stocked with all the furniture that he is likely to use, and the rest he can put away in the lumber room of his library, where he can get it if he wants it"

According to Alzheimer's Research UK, those who exercise regularly and make exercise a part of their lifestyle lower their risks of Alzheimer's disease.

Dementia is a global problem that currently sees a diagnosis every four seconds, with an estimated 115 million predicted to suffer from some type of dementia disorder by the year 2050.

Harvard Medical School reports that exercise has numerous benefits for the brain.

One study conducted at the University of British Columbia concluded that regular aerobic exercise, balance training, and muscle and resistance workouts seem to increase the size of the hippocampus, the part of the brain that regulates learning and verbal memory.

Exercise also helps to increase oxygen levels in the brain, which helps to improve mental performance, slow rate of fatigue, improves overall brain function, enhances motor skills, and stimulates better blood flow throughout the body. Oxygen and blood flow are lifelines of the human brain.

Exercise Works For The Brain In Two Key Ways
Directly

· Reduces insulin resistance
· Reduces inflammation
· Stimulates the release of growth factors that promote brain cell health
· Promotes new blood vessel growth
· Supports growth and survival of new brain cells

Indirectly, exercise deals with problems that contribute to various levels of cognitive impairment

· Boosts mood
· Provides for better sleep
· Reduces stress
· Lowers anxiety

Harvard Medical School reports that numerous studies have suggested that the prefrontal cortex and the medial temporal cortex, both parts of the brain that control memory and thinking are larger in volume in people who regularly exercise than in people who do not.

The good news is that aerobic exercise is not only good for the brain but for the body, specifically the heart, and reducing risks for overweight or obesity, which lead to a host of other health problems and even premature death.

Don't forget strength training, as lifting weights, using resistance bands and doing bodyweight exercises seriously boosts brain power, improves mood, trains decision making skills and enhances concentration.

Mind-Body Exercises

Yoga, Tai Chi and Qigong are forms of mind-body exercise that not only work the body, but also specifically utilize the mind in their movements and poses.

· One of their greatest benefits of mind-body exercise is the calming of the mind, where in quiet, mental and brain health is significantly improved

· Improve blood circulation to the brain

· Builds focus and memory skills

· Reduce stress

· Teaches controlled breathing to reduce anxiety

· Helps manage and prevent depression

· Strengthens the ability to focus and concentrate not only during the exercise session, but through the training becomes a skill that you can use in all other parts of your life

Two main groups of minerals and vitamins are essentially for the health of the brain. You may be surprised to learn that many people, even those living in developed countries like the US, are failing to get sufficient amounts of these nutrients.

English researchers completed a meta-analysis of 20 years' worth of trials and reviews to identify those nutrients that do the most for regulating brain health.

They discovered that vitamin C, the B complex vitamins, as well as magnesium, zinc, and calcium have the greatest relevance to brain health.

Nutrients are thought to affect the brain in four different ways.

· The B and C complex vitamins work together and produce neurotransmitters for the central nervous system.

· The B complex vitamins assist in quick and accurate neurotransmitter signals.

· Both of these groups of nutrients assist in converting food into the molecules required for fueling brain cells.

· The B complex vitamins reduce homocysteine levels, which is indicative of inflammation, increasing the risk of blood vessel diseases.

While the brain only accounts for around three percent of the body's total weight, it devours as much as 25% of blood glucose while the body is resting. Additionally, within the body brain tissue contains the highest levels of vitamin C.

We know that our bodies only store small amounts of water-soluble vitamins and minerals, such as vitamins C and the B complex, zinc, and magnesium. People who lead demanding lives, and the elderly, are in need of additional nutrients if they wish to maintain optimal levels of brain function.

Vitamin C

Vitamin C is a powerful antioxidant that plays a key role in healthy brain function, reduces the risk of stroke, and serves as a regulator for more than a dozen neurochemicals.

Vitamin C Foods: Tomatoes, citrus fruits – lemons, oranges and grapefruits

• B6. A vitamin B6 deficiency can result in memory loss and depression, so it's vital to consume enough B6 to keep your mind and memory sharp.

Vitamin B6 Foods: fish, beef liver, starchy vegetables (potatoes, corn), fruit (expect citrus), B6 fortified cereals and poultry

• B12. Vitamin B12 is vital for neuro health, and is responsible for producing the sheath that protects the nerves. A vitamin B12 deficiency causes the sheath to expose nerves, which results in pain and neuropathy.

Animal foods are the only natural source of vitamin B12: red meat, poultry, and dairy products – milk and cheese and eggs.

• **B1** - Thiamine is a mood booster, and can prevent depression and well as improve overall mood. It plays an important role in creating enzymes and amino acids.

Food sources of B1: liver, beef, oats, oranges, pork, eggs, seeds, legumes, dried milk, peas and yeast and fortified foods such as rice, pasta, breads, cereals and flour.

• **B2** - Riboflavin handles the transmission of impulses. A deficiency can result in migraines, epilepsy, MS, and an increased risk of dementia.

• **Foods sources of B2:** Lamb, beef livers, yogurt, milk, mushrooms, spinach, almonds, sun-dried tomatoes, salmon, and eggs.

• **B3** - Niacin is known for reducing cholesterol, and it also stimulates the brain.

Foods sources of B3: turkey, chicken, peanuts, mushrooms, liver, tuna, green peas, grass-fed beef, sunflower seeds, and avocados.

· **B9** - Folate or folic acid helps to reduce homocysteine levels within the brain. This reduces the risk of dementia, and it can also slow down the progression of the disease for those who are already suffering from a type of dementia. It works to protect the brain from stress.

Foods rich in folate: spinach, all greens, asparagus, oranges, broccoli, papaya, grapefruit, grapes, bananas, cantaloupes, strawberries, beans, peas, and lentils, okra, avocado, seeds and nuts, okra, cauliflower, beets, corn, celery, carrots and squash.

Vitamins For The Brain

The best way to get the necessary vitamins and nutrients that your body and brain need for optimal function is through a healthy diet. If you are enjoying a healthy diet, there shouldn't be a need for supplements. However, this is not always possible for everyone. Whether you have allergies, or you are a vegetarian of vegan, you may be lacking in certain supplements and losing out on boosting your brain health.

- Magnesium is a common deficiency, so a 200mg supplement twice a day may be beneficial to you.

- Vitamin C is water soluble, so your body requires replenishment. A 250mg supplement every day is a safe place to start.

- B complex. You can find a general B complex vitamin and one every day is sufficient.

WebMD reports that the Mediterranean diet, which is rich in whole grains, olive oil, fish, nuts, and green leafy vegetables not only supports brain health throughout life, but also reduces risks for Alzheimer's disease.

Numerous spices and herbs, including ginger, cinnamon, and turmeric contain key antioxidants that help lower levels of harmful inflammation.

Many bright colored fruits and vegetables, such as leafy greens, tomatoes, citrus fruit, and berries also contain key antioxidants that support brain health and help reduce oxidative stress that leads to premature aging.

· One cup of coffee has more antioxidants than a standard serving of raspberries, oranges, grape juice, and even blueberries that help reduce inflammation (National Center for Complementary and Integrative Health).

· The National Institute of Health report that thanks to the antioxidants in coffee, those who drink four cups of coffee a day are around 10% less likely to be affected by depression as compared to those who do not drink it.

· Coffee has been shown in numerous studies to lower risks for dementia, and improve memory.

· One study found a 40% reduction in brain cancer in both men and women. (Holick, et al, published on The American Association For Cancer Research).

· Studies published in The Journal of American Medical Association found caffeine to reduce the risks of developing Parkinson's disease by 60%.

· Studies from Portugal's Porto University Medical School found coffee to lower risks of Alzheimer's by as much as 65%.

· Caffeine works in the brain to increase dopamine levels, helping to firing those neurons that boost mood, focus, and concentration.

· A lot of research has found it to increase attention span, improve logical thinking and reaction time.

· Studies from Université de Nancy, found coffee to improve memory, vigilance, and cognitive function.

· Coffee boosts those brain chemicals, which promote wellbeing.

· A study from South Korea's Seoul National University showed that just the smell of coffee could actually reduce the effects of stress that results from sleep deprivation. Your nose knows a good thing when it smells it, and coffee is no exception.

· The Mayo Clinic states that 100% pure green and black teas contain key antioxidants that support brain health and cognitive function.

The Alzheimer's Association and other authorities report that diabetes, obesity, depression, high cholesterol, high blood pressure and other chronic conditions increase risks of dementia.

Lifestyle choices more often than not dictate whether you suffer from these conditions or no, inducing, diet, exercise, and stress control. Consider your lifestyle and make all necessary changes as soon as possible.

Talk to your doctor to prevent these harmful conditions and make sure to get regular check-ups, blood tests, and age appropriate screenings.

Risk: Obesity and Diabetes

· Change your eating habits and practice moderation and portion control
· Reduce or eliminate intake of simple carbs, sugars and white starches
· Eliminate junk food
· Eat lean protein
· Eat healthy fats, fish, nuts and avocados
· Eat more fiber
· Exercise for at least 30 minutes 5 times a week

Risk: Hypertension

High blood pressure causes structural damage in the brain that can lead to mental decline.

· Eat less salt
· Keep your blood pressure under 120/80 mmHg
· Monitor your blood pressure regularly
· Exercise for at least 30 minutes 5 times a week
· Maintain a healthy weight

Risk: Heart Disease and High Cholesterol

· Eat a healthy diet
· Exercise regularly
· Get age-appropriate health screenings
· Assess your individual risks with your doctor
· Follow doctor's orders

Mental

The Human Mind: Use It Or Lose It

Exercise for your mind, is just as critical as exercise for the body. Think of it as a muscle that will shrink and lose its strength when it is not being used and trained.

The brain is a dynamic organ, learning, thinking and using it help to improve its functioning and promotes new neuron growth, which incidentally helps prevent dementia from developing and keeps it strong and vital.

Build Your Cognitive Reserve

Harvard Medical School reports that one of the key concepts in understanding cognitive health is cognitive reserve. **Cognitive reserve is the brain's ability to improvise and identify alternate ways of getting something done.** This phenomenon allows the brain to change how it operates with available recourses aiding in dealing with challenges.

The concept of cognitive reserve dates back to the 1980s, when researchers noted people who lacked any dementia symptoms but whose brains at autopsy showed brain changes seen with advanced Alzheimer's disease. These people showed no symptoms because they had a big enough cognitive reserve, which helped to offset the typical damage done by Alzheimer's and therefore their brains continued to function normally.

> "Dr. Einstein was not successful in school, but he found something in the air from his own imagination and his own brain power, and look what he did"
>
> *Eartha Kitt*

Since that time, research has shown that those who have a greater cognitive reserve are less likely to develop degenerative brain changes, such as those seen with dementia, stroke, and Parkinson's disease.

A strong cognitive reserve also promotes better functioning through taxing situations, such as stressful situations, a car accident, or even environmental toxins. These types of scenarios are more taxing to the brain and require extra effort, and when the brain lacks in coping skills, confusion, delirium and signs of disease can occur.

Cognitive reserve begins to develop in childhood but gest stronger as you age into adulthood. One of the most important tasks in maintaining a high level of brain and mental health is to sustain and support cognitive reserve.

It is developed and improved through a lifetime of curiosity, education, learning, embracing new activities, and developing new skills, all of which help the brain deal much more effectively with any and all failures and declines it may face.

"Use it or lose it" has never been truer.

"Any man who reads too much and uses his own brain too little falls into lazy habits of thinking"

Key ways to build your cognitive reserve include

· **Challenge the mind** with new never before done activities. Shlomo Breznitz, Ph.D., founder of Cognifit, and co-author of Maximum Brainpower: Challenging the Brain for Health and Wisdom believes that searching out new ways to engage your mind is the best way to stave off mental decline because it builds cognitive reserve.

· **Learn a new skill** that requires higher functioning, such as problem solving, for example, learn to plumb your sink or build something from scratch. The more confusing the skill the better, as it provides a higher challenge for the mind and forces your brain out of novelty and into variety, making it respond to new and challenging information and stimuli.

· **Critical thinking challenges the brain**, a college English writing class is a great way to challenge yourself in this area

· **Challenge weaknesses** – Battle brain routine and engage yourself in activities where you have weakness. If for example, you have never done any home improvement, choose a project and get started. If writing has challenged you in the past, start writing your life story.

· **Start using your non-dominant hand** – if you're right handed, use your left hand, and vice versa.

· **Get a degree**

· **Travel** to new and never before seen places

· **Learn a new language**

· **Learn a musical instrument**

· **Paint or sculpt**

In short, do things you have never done before, the experience, and learning process will stimulate cognitive reserve. Breznitz says, "Challenging the brain helps maintain cognitive vigor and capacity. And maintaining our cognitive health maintains our quality of life."

Meditation just maybe one of the most significant and miraculous activities for the health of your brain and overall mental fitness.

Anti-Aging

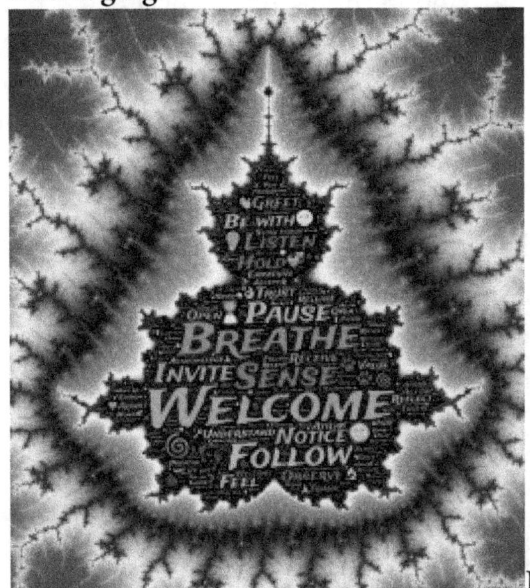

In 2015, researchers from UCLA published findings in Frontiers in Psychology that fund aging subjects who meditated had better-preserved brains than those who never mediated. Specifically, those who subjects who engaged in meditation for about 20 years actually had a widespread increase in volumes of gray matter in the brain.

The study's author, Florian Kurth, notes, *We expected rather small and"distinct effects located in some of the regions that had previously been associated with meditating. Instead, what we actually observed was a widespread effect of meditation "that encompassed regions throughout the entire brain*

Actual Brain Structure Changes

A 2011 Harvard study (Lazar, et al) found that mindfulness meditation actually changes brain structure. Specifically, the model subjects used was eight weeks of Mindfulness-Based Stress Reduction (MBSR, developed by Jon Kabat-Zinn at the University of Massachusetts' Center for Mindfulness), which increased cortical thickness in the hippocampus, an area of the brain that controls memory, and learning. The study's senior author Sara Lazar notes, *This" study demonstrates that changes in brain structure may underlie some of these reported improvements and that people are not just feeling better because they are "spending time relaxing*

Additionally, decreases in brain cell volumes in the amygdala were seen, and since the amygdala controls stress, anxiety, and fear reactions, this means significant benefits for brain, physical, emotional, and mental health.

The changes observed by researchers were confirmed by study subjects who reported changes in stress levels. In a follow-up study with the same subjects, positive changes in areas of the brain linked to mood and arousal were observed after meditation training, with study subjects reporting improvements in psychological well-being.

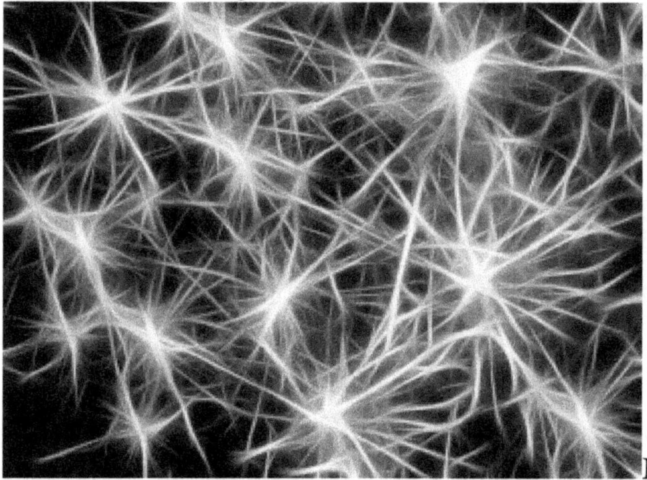

Britta Hölzel, first author of the paper and a research fellow at MGH and Giessen University in Germany says, *It is fascinating to see the brain's plasticity and that, by practicing" meditation, we can play an active role in changing the brain and can increase our "well-being and quality of life*

Improved Focus, Concentration, and Attention

Better focus, attention, and concentration skills are central to meditation, and may be its greatest gifts. Numerous studies have shown meditation to have significant effects on these three key areas of mental wellness and brain health.

Typically, these effects show very quickly and after just a few sessions of meditation, exemplifying how meditation is an effective form of brain training that's cognitive benefits are seen long after any specific meditation is over.

Stops Mind Wandering

Yale University discovered that mindfulness meditation reduces activity in the DMN (default mode network), the area responsible for mind wandering.

Mind wandering is associated with excessive worry, and dampening of overall happiness. This is the difference between a quiet and calm mind, and one that is frenzied and filled with worry. In fact, numerous studies have shown meditation to be incredibly effective at quieting the mind, and therefore reducing activity in the DMN.

Depression

Meditation has effects that are similar to medications used for both anxiety and depression.

A 2014 review study conducted by Johns Hopkins examined the relationship between mindfulness meditation and its effect on anxiety and depression. The findings concluded that mediation, which is an active form of brain training, is a key tool in managing depression.

Reduces Anxiety

Numerous studies have shown, and many meditators will attest to meditation's positive effects on anxiety levels. MBSR has been shown effective in this regard with significant and long lasting changes.

Research has also shown mindfulness meditation, as opposed to breath meditation practices, to also greatly reduce anxiety. In this proactive, brain changes are mediated through regions that regulate "me-centered) thoughts.

Getting Started

Meditation offers numerous benefits for the brain and mental health, but in order to maintain these, you must practice daily, and be vigilant or else the brain can easily revert to its old ways. Whenever possible, it is best to get a meditation mentor or trainer to benefit from this amazing ancient practice.

Experts agree that games and puzzles are perfect exercises for your brain. Whether you choose crosswords, Sudoku, chess, brain game apps, brain teasers or even video games your brain will benefit from the experience.

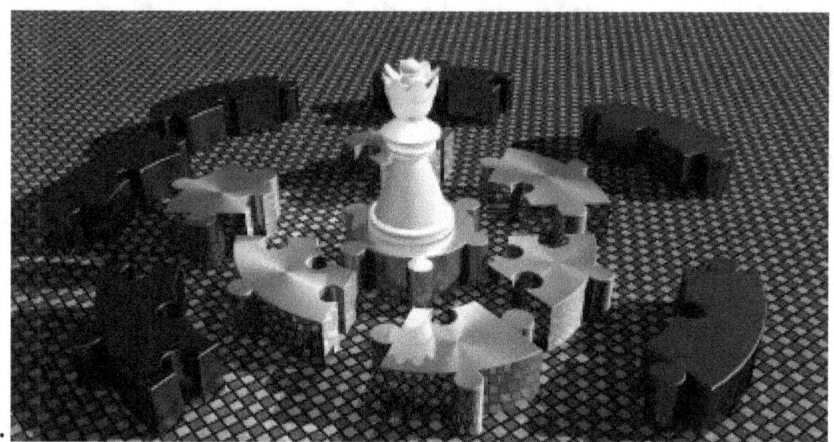

Stimulate the mind
- Promote logical thinking
- Learn new skills
- Hone concentration skills
- Improve mood
- Feelings of accomplishment
- Boost Focus Skills
- May slow degeneration in brain-degenerative disease
- May delay memory loss of dementia
- Exercise critical thinking skills
- Hone problem solving skills

Emotional And Lifestyle

Happiness and positivity are key to the health of your brain. Pleasure can stimulate your brain, priming it to respond to further reinforce pleasure. Your brain is essentially rewarding you in a way that should steer you to happiness. You can return the favor by giving it rewards to encourage it to keep on fine-tuning.

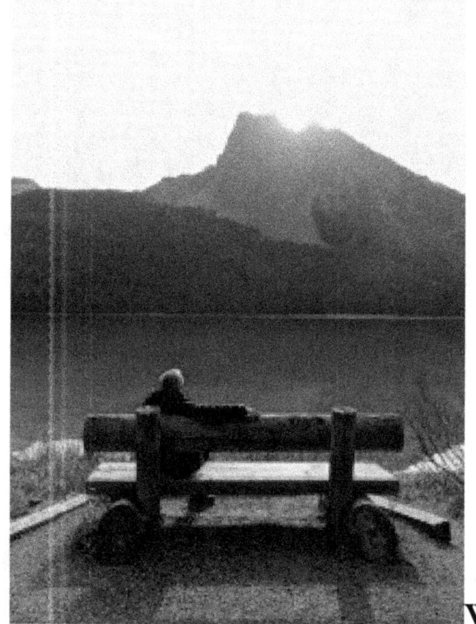

Why would you want to be happy? Well, aside from the fact that you'll be fun to hang out with:

· Happiness stimulates nerve connection growth.

· Happiness boosts cognitive abilities, thus increasing productivity.

· Happiness increases your ability to think logically and analyze.

· Happiness spurs happier thoughts.

· Happiness has an impact on how you see your surroundings.

· Happiness improves concentration.

· Happy people are often quick to solve problems, mentally alert, and far more creative than their pessimistic counterparts are.

The Power of Positivity

Thoughts form who you are as a person, thus how you face the world. Those thoughts dictate how far you will go spiritually, physically, and mentally. Your inner voice is often a reflection of external circumstances.

Every thought that you have, though, releases chemicals in the brain. When your brain is focused on the negative, it is sapped of its positivity. This causes your brain to slow down, and not only will it affect the brain's ability to function, it can also lead to mental health problems.

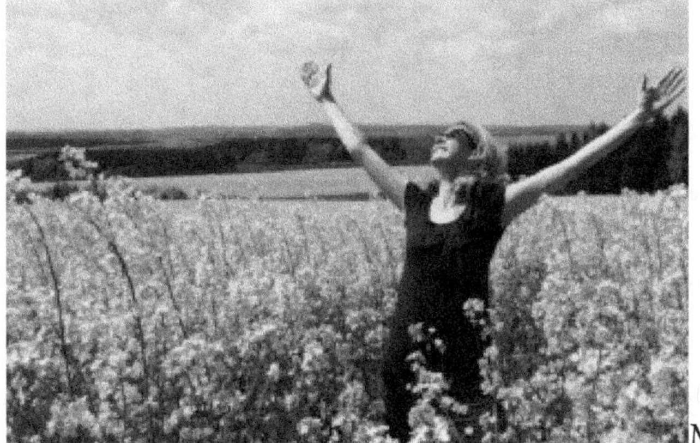

Meanwhile, positive thoughts produce serotonin and decrease levels of cortisol. This produces a sense of well-being, and encourages your brain to function at capacity. Positive thinking and happiness support the growth of your brain, and also generate and reinforce new synapses. This is especially true of the prefrontal cortex region of the brain, and this is the region, which acts as an integration center for the best of your brain functions.

This isn't just regulating signals the brain, but also to your body, allowing you to consider what you are doing physically. The prefrontal cortex provides control over emotional responses and provides you with the ability to focus on things of your choosing.

Why Positivity Brings Happiness

Neuroscientists have found people with a cheerful outlook are more likely to be optimistic. This is due to high levels of activity in the prefrontal cortex. It isn't just the neuroscientists who have discovered this; behavioral scientists have found the same thing.

Furthermore, optimists show higher cognitive functional, as well as high levels of motivation, and emotional control. The optimist keeps better moods, leading to greater physical health, driving perseverance, and success.

The positive thinkers and optimists among us:

· Enjoy strong relationships

· Lead lives that are rich and fulfilled

· Enjoy longer lives

· Have healthy habits

· Are more social

· Have strong immune systems

· While optimists take control of their lives and responsibility for those actions, the pessimist tends to look at negative events as a permanent problem, with positive events being a passing phase.

The negative thinkers and pessimists among us:

· Are more likely to suffer from depression
· Don't perform as well in school or at work
· Have a shorter lifespan
· Struggle in personal relationships

The pessimist will compare themselves to everyone else around them, while the optimist doesn't indulge in comparisons. If you are a pessimist, there's good news.

You can train your brain to rid yourself of negativity and turn your thoughts to positivity, thus inviting brain health and happiness to your life. Even those with a genetic predisposition to mental health issues can reduce its reoccurrence and impact by learning to turn negative thoughts into positive ones.

Negativity Breeds Imbalance

Thinking negatively can make it difficult to process your thoughts and find solutions to problems you face. Feeling scared (which is common for people focused on the negative) decreases cerebellum activity, thus slowing down the brain's ability to process information.

This has a direct impact on your ability to solve problems. In addition, it can have an impact on memory, impulse control, and mood.

5 Ways To Refocus Your Thinking

It really takes practice to rewire your brain to think in a positive manner, versus a negative one, especially if negativity is deeply engrained. However, practice really does make perfect in this case.

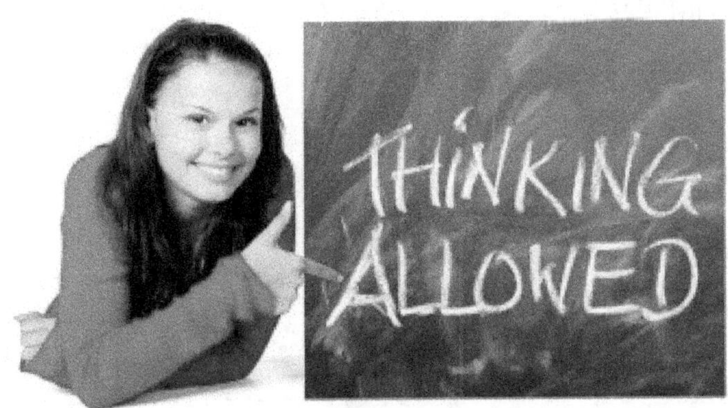

As you work to eliminate negative thoughts from your life, you will fail, and will not always be able to think in a positive manner, but the more you practice the easier it will get, as it becomes habitual, instead of a forced effort.

Positive thinking will not be achieved over night, but taking it one day at a time is the best way to learn this type of thought process.

Yes, I Can

Believing in yourself is a good place to start, as often some of the most negative thoughts we have are about ourselves.

For example, instead of "I know I can't cook this meal, like mom does," change that to "I know I can cook this meal and make it great." As you have other "I can't" statements pop up in your head, change them to "I cans."

Track Negativity

Become aware and note when you are most negative. Is it during stressful days? During work? When you are around your spouse?

Pinpointing reasons or triggers for negativity allows you to take action to become more positive about the situation.

Affirmations

Affirmations can help you get in the practice of positive thinking since they are always stated in the present as if the action or thing that is being affirmed has already happened or is assumed to be true. **Self-affirmation is defined as an act demonstrating one's adequacy. Any action that affirms our core value can act as a self-affirmation.**

Affirmations are by definition positive and can therefore help you reprogram your mind towards positivity.

For example

- I am smart
- I am an optimist
- I am self-driven
- I know how to solve problems
- I am having a great day
- Today, is a positive day in my life
- I am a great cook
- I love life and everyday that comes with it

Start & Finish Your Day With Affirmations

Begin your day with a positive affirmation; remind yourself that the day is filled with opportunities. Create an affirmation that will leave you feeling great and set you up to face your day. Make it part of your morning routine, as your mind is clear from sleep and ready to be set up for the day.

It's helpful to repeat this process in the evening as your mind can focus on these goals subconsciously as you sleep.

Of course, there are numerous opportunities during the day for affirmations as well, and phone apps that can help you with this process.

Spend Time With Positive People

One of the greatest ways to learn positivity is to spend time with optimists, as they have the amazing ability to see the silver lining behind every cloud. They are a true-life example of positive thinking and you can learn a lot by watching them in action.

You've likely heard it more times, than you can remember- laughter is the best medicine. This is true in many respects, as laughter can bring about meaningful neurochemical and physiological changes that can benefit the body.

In particular, laughter can improve brain health, and help manage many "silent" disorders, not easily observed by medical practitioners, or society as a whole.

· Laughter boosts creativity as humor and creativity share a similar part of the brain.

· Improves executive function by allowing the brain to improve its delegating work.

· Laughter relieves stress and a reduction in stress hormones improves brain function.

· Alzheimer's and Parkinson's are associated with dopamine dysfunction, and laughter stimulates dopamine release inside the brain.

· The most sought after anti-aging hormone in the body, the growth hormone, is boosted significantly by laughter, so you can literally add years to your life by laughing more often.

· Inflammation is what ultimately leads to breakdown of body processes and promotes aging, causing a range of diseases including but not limited to cancer and brain degenerative conditions. Laughter exerts an anti-inflammatory effect, reducing risk of developing cancers, cardiovascular disease, and degenerative diseases of the brain.

So laugh more often! Seek out opportunists for laughter, such as going to comedy clubs, or even placing a joke of the day calendar on your desk, your brain will thank you for it.

> **FACT**
> Sleep deprivation
> can impair
> judgment and
> slow reaction

WebMd reports that sleep is critical for the health of your brain and day to day functioning. Getting a good night's sleep on a regular basis improves mood, supports healthy immune system functioning, and may reduce concentrations of beta-amyloid plaque, an abnormal protein that develops in the brain and is linked to Alzheimer's disease.

Socializing And Human Connections

The Alzheimer's Association advises that leading an active social life protects against memory loss. Spending time with friends and family and engaging in stimulating conversation supports overall brain health and promotes mental wellness. Get involved in the community; hobby clubs are a great way to meet new people that share your interests.

Having a healthy social life also helps prevent and combat depression and boosts intellectual stimulation. Numerous studies have indicated that people who enjoyed a rich social life have the slowest rate of memory decline.

Get A Pet

Having a pet can go a long way to boosting your mental and emotional health. Unconditional love is their unique gift to humans, along with their ability to calm us down, boost immunity and heart health, and enhance our social lives, along with promoting fun, play, and opportunities for laughter.

> **FACT**
> **The smell of chocolate increases theta brain waves, which**

An article by Semantic Scholar details popular methods of reducing anxiety, and inducing relaxation, one of which is Biofeedback.

"Biofeedback is one of the most useful adjuncts in treating physiologic hyperarousal-both episodic and chronic-seen in anxiety disorders. It has also proved helpful for patients who are learning to reduce fearful anticipation triggers through cognitive/behavior therapies."

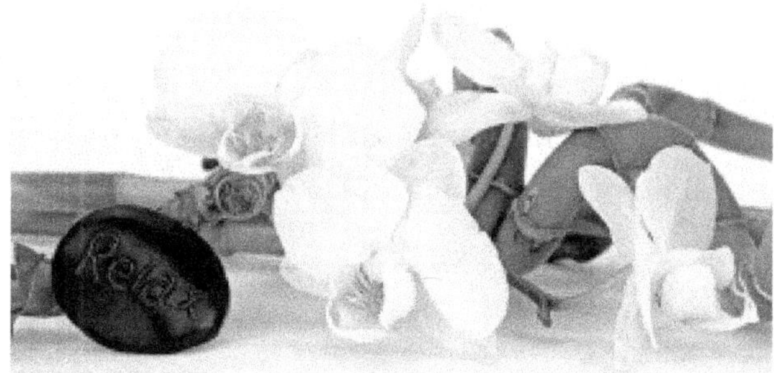

Different things relax different people. For example, while silence affords some the opportunity to peacefully reflect, music can accomplish the same purpose for other. Each of us is familiar with what does and does not have a calming effect on our minds.

The key is to make calming influences a priority, recognizing the importance of facilitating an environment in which our respective brains can thrive.

Mind-body exercises, including meditation and yoga help reduce stress and elicit the relaxation response in the body, which helps reduce levels of the stress hormone cortisol.

Furthermore, both practices offer numerous mental, emotional, and physical health benefits, helping you to be more well overall, which in turn supports brain health.

Physical health is often dictated by mental health, so it is imperative to remain committed to mental health. This modern era of incessant texts, calls, emails, and social media updates do not make it easy, but breaking away from it to allow our brains to breathe, so to speak, and must be as much a part of one's schedule as those deadlines and to-do lists.

Whatever means you find most helpful, relaxation, both mental and physical, is paramount to brain health and mental wellness.

> **FACT**
> Chronic stress affects focus, concentration, memory, learning abilities and leads to brain burnout that may render you unable to perform in your daily life

Stress and cortisol aren't just having a serious impact on the body; it's equally as dangerous to the brain. Some of the symptoms are common, so you're likely to be familiar with stress causing worry, anxiety, and memory issues. However, many of the effects that stress is having on the brain are considered behind the scenes problems. You won't notice that they're happening to you, but eventually you start to pick up on their side effects.

Stress Leads To Brain Cell Killing Free Radicals

Free radicals attack brain cells just as oxygen does to metal, resulting in rust. They actively punch holes in the walls of your brain cells, resulting in ruptures and the ultimate death of the brain cell. It doesn't help that stress often prompts sufferers to eat more junk food, drink excessively, and eat fatty foods- all of these increase the free radical load.

Over Emotional And Forgetful

The first sign that you may pick up on will be the memory problems. You'll forget appointments, lose your keys, and scramble for the most basic memory. This only serves to compound stress. This often results in difficulty controlling your emotions, too. While the signals of the brain that associated with memories will be weakened by stress, those associated with your emotions only get stronger.

Anxiety And Fear

The amygdala is the fear center of the brain and this is where stress accumulates. High levels of cortisol will increase the activity in the amygdala, as well as its size, and the number of connections. This results in you feeling more fearful, fueling the cycle of stress, anxiety, and fear.

Stupidity

Yes, chronic stress *will* make you stupid. Think about the times where you have felt most stressed out. It's often when you're speaking in front of a crowd, in the middle of an exam, or sitting across from a prospective boss in a job interview. Suddenly stress kicks in and your brain freezes.

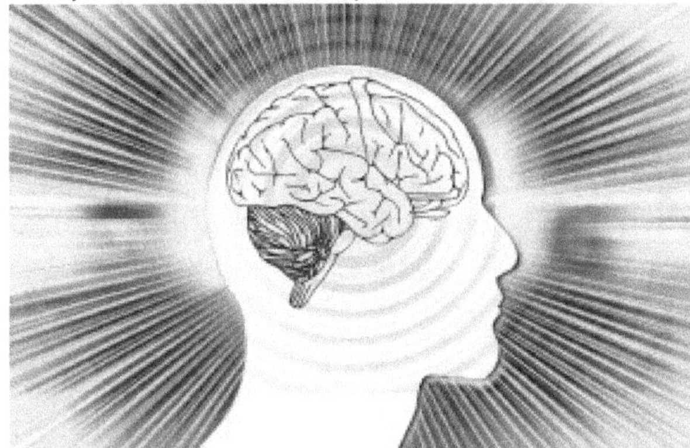

This is a throwback to evolution, with that fight or flight response. Unfortunately, we don't have much need for that, as we don't often face being chased down and eaten by the wildlife. The point is, stress can impair your memory, make it difficult for you to analyze data, and make decision making impossible to handle.

Mental Health

Neurotransmitters carry communication between brain cells, unfortunately, when suffering with chronic stress; neurotransmitters aren't being produced at the correct levels. This is particularly true of dopamine and serotonin. This can lead to depression, and it can also increase your risk and likelihood of addiction.

For women with low serotonin levels there is an increased risk of binge eating, anxiety, and depression. For men, the risks are impulse control disorders and alcoholism. Low levels of dopamine can result in depression, lethargy, and a lack of focus and motivation. In turn, people turn to sugar, drugs, caffeine, and alcohol to boost dopamine levels, even temporarily.

Brain Shrinkage

Yes, stress can shrink your brain, measurably so. An increase in cortisol levels doesn't just *stop* new neurons from being generated in the hippocampus; it can also shrink and kill them. The hippocampus is crucial in emotional regulation, as well as stored memory and learning. Additionally, chronic stress can shrink the prefrontal cortex, which controls impulse behavior, decision making, and working memory.

Neurodegenerative Diseases

This could be one of the most worrying results when it comes to chronic stress and brain health. It increases the risk of Alzheimer's and dementia. For Americans, Alzheimer's is sixth on the table when it comes to causes of death. One in three American seniors will die because of some form of dementia. While there may not be a cure, what we do know is that stress steeply increases the risk of dementia.

As you can see from the above, effectively managing stress is crucial to the health of your brain and your overall mental wellness.

There are many ways to manage stress and keep it from affecting your health.

1. Exercise of any kind
2. Stretching

1. Tai chi

1. Yoga
2. Meditation
3. Take a warm bath
4. Give yourself a scalp massage
5. Swedish massage
6. Aromatherapy, and especially lavender essential oils induce calm and melt away stress
7. Spa days
8. Guided imagery
9. Self-hypnosis
10. Learn autogenic, a practice that teaches you to relax your body on command
11. Progressive muscle relaxation
12. Deep breathing
13. Gardening
14. Take regular breaks
15. Establish a routine
16. Identify what is causing you stress and do everything possible to eliminate those things whenever possible
17. Get out of unhealthy relationships
18. Focus on one worry at a time
19. Stop multi-tasking
20. Delegate
21. Stop trying to control everything and let go that which you cannot change

22. Prioritize and stop overwhelming yourself
23. Don't victimize yourself by accepting that stress is normal due to your job or any other reason, this normalizes stress which deters you from addressing it appropriately
24. Take a vacation
25. Get a hobby that you love
26. Be present and practice mindfulness, which will help you focus on only the present moment
27. Be grateful for all you have and stop dwelling on the negatives
28. Stop procrastinating
29. Keep a journal
30. Eat a well-balanced and nutritious diet
31. Listen to music
32. Play music
33. Hone your time management skills
34. Clean your house, sometimes physical labor really lowers stress levels and the absence of a mess and clutter helps calm you
35. Get enough sleep
36. Invest in a stress ball
37. Visualize calm
38. Laugh often
39. Count to ten at times of stress and take a time out away from the situation to restart your frame of mind
40. Try to see the positive in all situations, positive thinkers are much better at handling stress than negative thinkers and pessimists
41. Make time for you every day
42. Unplug
43. Rip paper – the action and noise paper makes when it is being ripped can help you to feel in control and powerful when you are stressed out and feel out of control.
44. Stay organized, clutter is havoc that spills over into your mindset
45. Act silly
46. See a stress management counselor or your doctor
47. Sip chamomile tea
48. Boost your vitamin and mineral intake

49. Avoid junk food
50. Lower your sugar intake as sugar spikes blood sugar levels causing you to crash and burn
51. Increase your magnesium intake as deficiencies induce stress
52. Have sex
53. Cuddle with your pet
54. Go outside into nature and breathe fresh air
55. Connect with others and socialize
56. Learn to say no, this avoids overwhelm that leads to stress
57. Avoid stressful situations

Use Your Imagination

When we are children growing up, our imagination is the key to an untold world and it remains important as you grow for its unique ability to improve brain health.

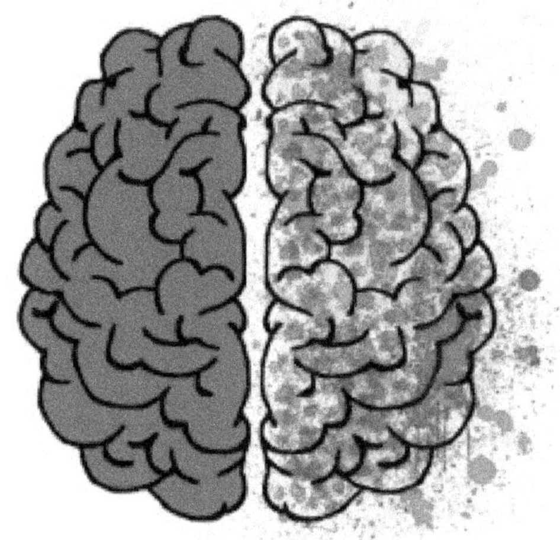

Imagination unleashes creativity, allowing you to live a life filled with potential. The creative individual does not see the sky as the limit, instead the limit is as far as he or she can imagine. They not only think outside the box, for them there is no box, and so their brains are constantly challenged, humming and conjuring up all sorts of goodies. Anything the mind can conjure is good enough to become true, be it work, life, personal goals accomplishments or anything else.

Having a more active imagination boosts empathy, the act of being truly sympathetic to another person's cause, without ever actually experiencing it yourself. Your imagination may leave you well poised to offer a shoulder for support, and being of service towards other people in that way, promotes your own mental health and emotional wellness.

Imagination forges stronger neuronal connections in the brain, which make you who you are, support memory functions and keep the brain vibrant, strong, and thriving.

Imagination promotes social interaction, as people with a more active imagination find it easier to relate and deal with people from all walks of life. Social interaction has been proven by scientific studies to reduce risks of dementia, and onset of age-related cognitive decline to keep the brain young, and thriving as you age.

The Alzheimer's Association advises that leading an active social life protects against memory loss. Spending time with friends and family and engaging in stimulating conversation supports overall brain health, forms new connections in the brain, and promotes mental wellness.

Cultivate and promote your own imagination whenever possible, your brain is counting on you!

Keeping Your Memory Healthy Throughout Aging

"My dull brain was wrought with things forgotten"

- William Shakespeare

We're all prone to a senior moment now and then, no matter the age. Whether it's forgetting where you left the keys, or going into a room and wondering what on earth, it is that you're doing there.

These memory lapses can happen at any age; however, aging is a contributing factor to memory loss. This is often compounded by neurological illnesses, organic disorders, and brain injuries.

However, not all is lost, there are plenty of which helps stave off cognitive decline to maintain healthy memory throughout aging.

· Eat a well-balanced diet and avoid trans fats entirely.

· Quit smoking and reduce alcohol intake to just one alcoholic beverage a day.

· Exercise regularly and stay active.

· Get at least seven hours of sleep every night.

· Maintain healthy and strong social connections.

There are varieties of health problems that can result in cognitive impairment; these include high cholesterol, high blood pressure, depression, diabetes, and sleep apnea. If you already have one of these conditions, it is imperative that you follow these guidelines strictly.

Thanks to many decades of research, we know have plenty of strategies that can help you keep your brain active and maintain your memory as you age.

Actively Learn

It doesn't matter how old you are, you can continue to learn. Keeping your brain challenged is an excellent way to stimulate your brain and maintain strong connections between brain cells. Even if you believe that your job is keeping your brain active, look for a hobby to further support brain function. Whether it's a book group, knitting circle, learning a new language, or tackling your life story. It's important to exercise your brain in different ways so that it doesn't fall into one strict pattern of thought.

Repeat To Remember

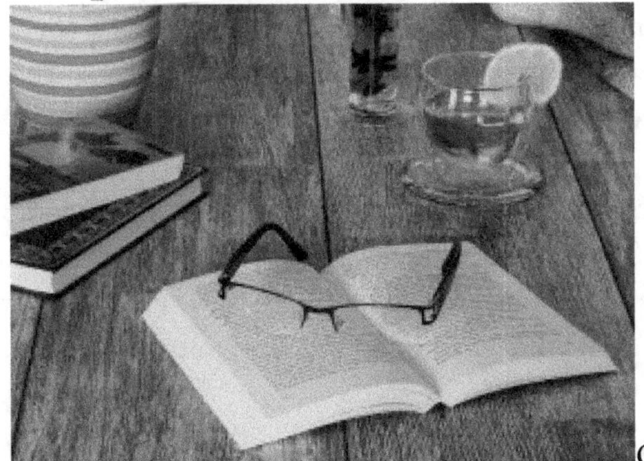

One of the most effective ways to retain information is by repeating it. Whether it's a thought that you've had, a piece of information that you have heard or read, take time out to write it down or say it aloud. This will reinforce the connection, thus improving the memory. A good example of this is when you meet someone new and they introduce themselves, repeat their name back as you greet them. You'll soon find that you'll remember the name of everyone you meet.

Economize

If you aren't wasting brain energy on recalling where you left your purse or keys, then you will be far better prepared to concentrate your brain power on learning and remembering new things.

Be smart, keep a calendar, write lists, and have important information handy so that you don't waste brain power thinking about things you can store outside of your brain. Have a place in your home that is designated for wallets, purses, and keys.

Space It Out

The most effective learning tool is repetition, which is when it is timed properly. Don't repeat something repeatedly within a short space of time. It isn't about cramming for finals. Start by repeating it initially and then again in an hour, and then in three hours, and then every day (this is assuming you're in need of retaining large amounts of information, for instance: a speech). It's far more effective to space this out, as it boosts recall.

Use Every Sense

The more senses you rely on when you are learning something, the more likely it is to stick in your memory. Consider what types of information you need to retain and couple them with smells and images. Even when the smell isn't present, your brain will be able to recall the information that accompanied it when required.

Don't be afraid to challenge every one of your senses when you're jumping into an unfamiliar situation. If you take up pottery, then don't just use your hands to feel, use your nose to take in the smell of the materials. If you take a cooking class, don't just pay attention to the smells or the tastes, take note of textures and sounds, too.

Dealing With Distractions

Distractions are everywhere, especially in the high-tech world we live in, with emails, text, social media updates, and apps coming at left and right.

Besides the external distractions, internal ones can also affect us, such as daydreaming, mind-wandering, and worrying.

When your attention is diverted in any way, you will lose concentration on the tasks in front of you.

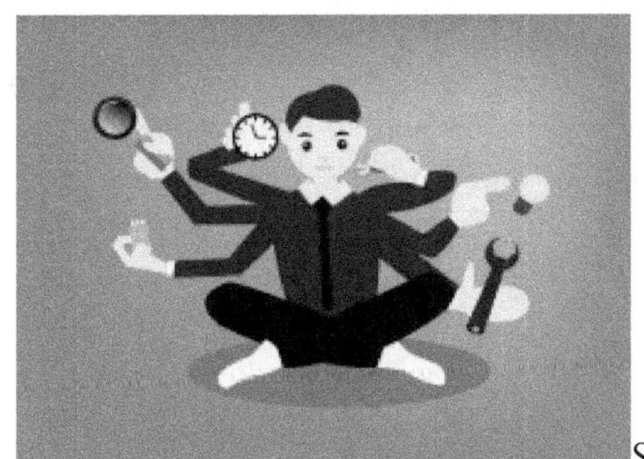

Studies prove that any type of distraction, can impact your short-term memory. The brain is a super computer, but even it can overloaded when attention is stretched over numerous things. Focus is necessary for memory retention, and it is difficult to focus when you are distracted.

The Problem With Multi-Tasking

Dr. Sanjay Gupta, neurosurgeon, associate chief of the neurosurgery service at Grady Memorial Hospital in Atlanta, Georgia and medical reporter for CNN reports that only 2% of the population is actually super multitaskers, and that multi-tasking is considered a genetic gift. Mostly, those who believe they are great multitaskers, are usually the worst.

A study published in Proceedings Of The National Academy Of Sciences, reports that multitasking actually makes you less productive as your brain only toggles back and forth from one task to another, which leads to losses in performances, learning, attention and short-term memory.

Issues With Multi-Tasking

· Diverts attention from one part of the brain to the other taking time, resources and brain cells

· Slows performance, affects quality of work and diminishes efficiency

· MRI scans show doing just two activities at once decreases attention by 37%

· Causes mental fatigue

· May possibly cause permanent cognitive damage

Concentration improves tremendously when we focus on just one thing at a time, and this can greatly improve your memory.

Potential Threats To Brain Health

> **"The chief function of the body is to carry the brain around"**
>
> *Thomas A. Edison*

Some medical conditions, including heart disease, hypertension, and diabetes can negatively affect your brain. Making smart lifestyle choices can prevent these conditions and therefore protect your brain.

Some medications, mixing alcohol with medications, and certain combinations of drugs can have an adverse effect on thinking and cognitive abilities. Speak with your doctor.

Drinking alcohol slows and impairs neuronal communication. It also results in memory loss, slurred speech, emotional chaos, and other short-term temporary effects. Long-term problems associated with excessive drinking, include, memory problems, cognitive impairment and emotional catastrophe.

Mood altering substances, such as illegal drugs, including but not limited to cocaine, heroin, and even prescription opiates can obviously have detrimental effects on the brain, including the killing of vital brain cells, loss of focus, concentration, motivation and many others.

Smoking increases risks for stroke. It also has an indirect effect on brain health as it greatly increases risks for heart disease.

Accidental brain injury can occur in older adults who have an increased risk for falls and other accidents.

Modern Lifestyle And Brain Health

> "Your conscious brain cannot multitask. If I'm speaking to you and checking my I-Phone at the same time, I'm doing neither. This is why our society is frazzled; this misconception that we can consciously do more than one thing at a time effectively"
>
> Deepak Chopra

An article published on Science Direct reports that humans are not getting smarter, in fact, *since the Victorian era,"* *"average IQs have gone down 1.6 points per decade for a total of 13.35 points*

A Trending Machine national poll published interesting results that millennials (those aged 18 to 34) are more forgetful than baby boomers, easily forgetting where they put their car keys or even what day it is.

Statistics Brain Statistics On Attention Spans

· The average attention span in 2000 was 12 seconds BUT only 8.25 seconds in 2015 (The average attention span of a gold fish is 9 seconds)

· 25% of teens forget major details of close friends and relatives

· 7% of people forget their own birthdays from time to time

· The average office worker checks his or her email 30 times per hour

Our brains are busier than ever before, and multi-tasking, which as previously mentioned is commonplace.

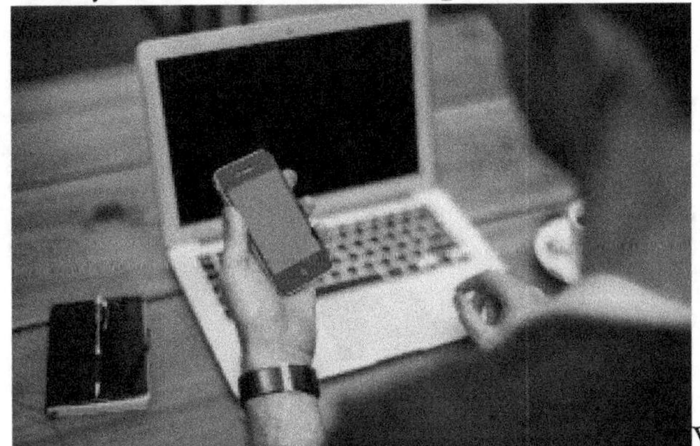We text while we're walking down the street, check email and social media while taking a business call, monitor social media updates, and have a YouTube video playing while doing homework or working and sit in our kitchens while making a shopping list on our smartphones, while listing to a podcast on how to plant perennials. Our phones are ringing, our email is pinging, and our brains are exhausted from attention darting back and forth from one thing to another.

Russ Poldrack, a neuroscientist at Stanford, discovered that learning while multitasking causes the newly learned information to go to the wrong part of the brain. Without distractions, the learned data goes where it should, to the hippocampus, where it is organized in numerous ways, making it easier to retrieve. Conversely, with multi-tasking the learned information goes to the striatum, a region of the brain that specializes in storing skills and procedures, not ideas and facts.

CNN Health reports that subjects who multitasked during cognitive tasks had significant IQ drops, as low as those seen after a missed night's sleep or after smoking marijuana.

Earl Miller, a neuroscientist at MIT (world expert on divided attention) says, *Our brains are not wired to multitask well... When people think they're"* *multitasking, they're actually just switching from one task to another very rapidly.* *"And every time they do, there's a cognitive cost in doing so*

Final Thoughts

> *"Every time you take in the good, you build a little bit of neural structure. Doing this a few times a day—for months and even years—will gradually change your brain, and how you feel and act, in far-reaching ways."* - Rick Hanson, Buddha's Brain: The Practical

• • • •

YOU HAVE A LOT OF CONTROL over the health of your brain and mental wellness. Making key lifestyle choices can go a long way to maintaining a high level of cognitive health and avoiding age-related cognitive decline.

The Cornerstones Of Holistic Brain Health

Physical

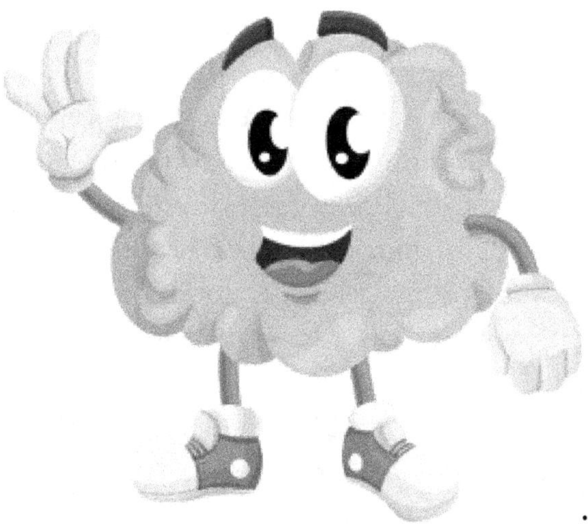

· Exercise

· Diet & Nutrition

· Medical Health

Mental

· Build Your Cognitive Reserve

· Meditation

· Games And Puzzles

Emotional And Lifestyle

- Happiness and Positivity
- Laughter
- Good Sleep
- Socializing And Human Connections
- Relaxation
- Stress Management

By following a healthy lifestyle and addressing these key areas of mental health, you can promote the health of your mind, and even possibly avoid age-related cognitive decline.

Stay well and take care!

| Page

Also by Danny Nandy

The Journey of Grief and Loss
Holistic Brain Health (6 Cornerstones of a Healthy Brain)
The Power of Choice
The Power of Positivity and Optimism
Master Your Destiny - The Anything Is Possible Mindset
Top 10 Lists - Life Lessons and Learning About You
The Complete Guide To Living A Balanced Lifestyle
The Power of Why - Push Your Motivation To New Limits